ENDORSEMENTS

This journal is going to be life-changing! As a trauma therapist, minister, and veteran, I know that the combination of spiritual, mental, and physical growth is vital for each one of us to find healing and freedom! Enjoy this 31-day journey to holistic health through the power of Scripture!

CLINT DAVIS, LPC, CSAT
clintdaviscounseling.com

Mental health can be an important part of our overall health, and with a growing number of people battling depression, anxiety, and more, it's important that we understand how we can maintain our own health and well-being. Mindi Foster has opened her heart to share her own story and to talk about a topic that countless people experience on a daily basis. However, what's fascinating is that she approaches the topic from an unconventional source, the Bible, and how it contains the understanding and strategies that will help you find hope, and mental and emotional wellness.

PAT CLARDY
Women's Ministry Leader

The Daily Dose reminds us that we are not alone in our challenges with our mind and heart. As a leader of diverse groups of people, this book is an important guide in understanding that many of us have mental health crises over our lifetimes, and that God has given us tools to guide us toward light. In this book, Foster sheds light on how we can look to Scripture for comfort and hope.

JENNIFER MCKINNEY
Executive Director, Mission 1:11

T0017091

Have you ever "bumped into" someone from your distant past and slowly come to realize that Jesus was most likely a part of that "bump"? Such was the case between myself and Mindi Foster. On a 90-minute Zoom interview, we dialogued about a lot of things—but most specifically, mental and emotional health from a Christian perspective. And as a leader who has dealt with significant clinical depression for the past 30 years of my life, I jumped into the dialogue wholeheartedly. I know firsthand how debilitating and isolating serious depression and anxiety can be. And so I'm authentically enthusiastic in my recommendation to you of Mindi's new book, *The Daily Dose.* In a Christian world too punctuated by "TRT" ("Typical Religious Talk"), Mindi's practical and tested suggestions give you a "play book" and strategies to push yourself gradually up from the dark pit that keeps trying to envelop you.

So happy reading! Grab a good cup of coffee, find a comfortable chair, and make this life-changing journey through Mindi Foster's *The Daily Dose.* Forfeit this opportunity at your own peril.

DR. JEANNE MAYO
International Speaker & Author
Founder & President, The Cadre
Founder & President, Youth Leader's Coach
Director, PREVAIL Women's Mastermind Cohort
Director, PLATINUM Leadership Coaching

The DAILY *Dose*

31 DAILY SUPPLEMENTS TO ENHANCE THE WAY YOU THINK

M. K. FOSTER

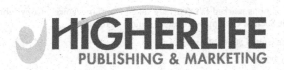

HIGHERLIFE
PUBLISHING & MARKETING

The Daily Dose

Published by HigherLife Development Services Inc.
PO Box 623307
Oviedo, Florida 32762
www.ahigherlife.com

CONTENTS

PREFACE

'M NOT A mental health professional or doctor, but this is my experience of many years of struggling with depression and suicide—even after my salvation at the age of seventeen. At the age of nineteen, I was training for ministry at a large church when I was diagnosed with depression. I was very angry, which is actually a major sign of depression. (I didn't say they were wrong; I was just distraught over it.)

The diagnosis came on my last appointment with no further help. No advice. No next steps. No supplemental resources. The psychologist just gave me her final thoughts and the diagnosis, then sent me on my way. I never saw that psychologist again.

Ministry didn't help matters. In fact, they complicated them. It was like waiting for a volcano to erupt. And it did, a few times.

I learned though. I didn't take medication (although I don't frown on it). I wasn't able to see another counselor either.

So, this is from someone who has learned as she has walked and often fought her way with God to get better. I've made some very bad decisions, but it did and does get better.

While writing this book, I lost a loved one to suicide. It

took the wind out of me and my family, not only because of his death, but because it was the second death in our family to suicide. I didn't think I could release this book because of what happened—but then I realized, how could I not?

So, this is for him and all the things I wish I would have told him in hope of helping him in his struggle.

This is for God.

This is for me.

This is for you and for anyone else that this might possibly help.

INTRODUCTION

TAKE YOUR VITAMINS

"Casting the whole of your care [all your anxieties, all your worries, all your concerns, once and for all] on Him, for He cares for you affectionately and cares about you watchfully."
(1 Peter 5:7 AMPC)

GOD REALLY CARES about *your* mental health! The Bible has a lot to say about the topic. Many themes in the Bible have to do with our thinking, like salvation, double-mindedness, pride (an issue of high-mindedness), humility (to be lowly of mind), strongholds (which are related to thought cycles), anxiety (a dividing of the mind), reasonings (how we process things in our minds), perceptions (the way we see things in our minds), imaginations (how we use creativity in our minds), etc.

Realizing how much the Bible speaks about our minds is important for two reasons:

1. If the Bible was written with so much information on the topic, then God knew about mental issues and gave us direction on how to handle them.
2. We cannot neglect Scripture in our quest for mental and emotional wellness.

The battle for mental health is so dangerous because it is one we cannot see. Disorders, anxieties, and diseases are an inside issue. Knowing this, God gave us the Holy Spirit to also do an inside job. He also gave us the Scriptures to help instruct and fortify our mental and emotional wellness.

Since I realized how much Scripture teaches about the mind, it has been a mission of mine to get people to understand these teachings. God does not care just for the world as a whole; He cares about *you*. The stress that impacts you, people who break your heart, the losses that have almost paralyzed you, the depression that has almost taken your life. . . . *He cares*. He cares so much that He has given you weapons to fight for your life.

This is not about how long you have been in church or how familiar you are with the Bible. This is about strategy. It's about application. It's about utilization.

These are all things that I've had to learn. I am passionate about mental and emotional wellness because of what God has done in and for me in these areas. You don't have to have a degree in psychology or the right medicine to be healthy.

I wrote *The Daily Dose* as a 31-day devotional to jump-start your focus on mental and emotional wellness. These devotionals are written to help "supplement" you as a vitamin would for your body. I offer tips and strategies that I've learned in hope that they will help you find wellness.

I want to invite you to join me for the next thirty-one days. Let's kick off a focus on strengthening and improving your mental and emotional wellness. I'll be praying for you.

Mindi

FIRST THINGS FIRST

"Now take the helmet of salvation . . ." (Ephesians 6:17)

THE FIRST STEP toward mental health is salvation. There are three different times that the "helmet of salvation" is mentioned in Scripture (1 Thessalonians 5:8 and Isaiah 59:17 are the other two). Contrary to popular belief, salvation is not just fire insurance to keep you from going to hell. There is actually so much more to the Good News that saves your soul. Health and wellness are your right as a Christian.

The Bible gives the idea that if you are going to win the battle of your mind, then salvation protects you like a helmet. Jesus did more than take on sin and shame to give us the confidence of eternal life. Salvation isn't just about giving us hope for eternity, but hope for life now.

Plainly put, your victory is declared through Him. You win the war, but you are still in the midst of battle, as Paul pictures here in Ephesians 6. This life is a battle regardless, so why not focus our efforts on the victory declared in Christ?

In combat, a person can survive injuries to the body, but a blow to the head could guarantee an advantage over the enemy. Your enemy, the devil, knows that. His lies take blow after blow at you, but that salvation helmet protects you. You may feel the power behind the strike, but the damage isn't as severe.

In order to get this helmet, salvation is the first step. If you have never asked Jesus to be your Savior, take a moment and ask Him into your heart. It's simple; just ask His forgiveness and for His help to truly know Him.

Now, with helmets on, let's kick-start a new journey.

"But we thank God for giving us the victory as conquerors through our Lord Jesus, the Anointed One."
(1 Corinthians 15:57 TPT)

FURTHER THOUGHTS

- Is your salvation just "fire insurance" to you? Why or why not?
- How can you utilize salvation as your "helmet" to protect you better?

A WEAPON MORE POWERFUL THAN PILLS

"For the word of God is living and active and full of power
[making it operative, energizing, and effective]. It is
sharper than any two-edged sword, penetrating as far as
the division of the soul and spirit [the completeness of a
person], and of both joints and marrow [the deepest parts
of our nature], exposing and judging the very thoughts and
intentions of the heart." (Hebrews 4:12 AMP)

WITH HELMETS IN hand (if you recall from yesterday), we are going to move forward for even more understanding of mental health and toxic thinking. With salvation guarding our heads, we have more than just a defensive strategy, but an offensive one too. Be ready to wield your swords for attack by utilizing Scripture.

It took me years to realize the potency of the Bible. It wasn't just poetic or even inspirational; it's absolutely powerful. The wisdom within the covers of Scripture is timeless, but it almost always takes consistency and time to garner the desired results (although I'd never rule out an instantaneous miracle).

If you're going to maximize the power that Scripture

offers, then upholding Scripture's authority and advice needs to be your priority. I'm not saying you should ditch your doctor and dump your pills, but trusting and relying on God and His Word is absolutely essential.

In order to learn how to think in a healthy manner, it is vital to understand that the Bible is God's thoughts for us. It is vital to base healthy thinking on what Scripture says in order to counter the thoughts and feelings that feed cycles of toxic thoughts and feelings.

Scripture has to be the ruler by which we measure every thought, habit, and opinion. If it doesn't line up with the truth, cut it off. Otherwise, you gamble with deception that will lead you into other issues that will never fulfill the best God has for you. It's simple, but it's far from easy.

From here forward, I pray that you will see your Bible differently. It's not a list of commands or some strange story from another time and culture, but instead, it is a powerful weapon that God intended for us to employ to take down the attacks of our enemy. This is not just a highly recommended idea here; your victory depends on how you wield your sword.

"And take the helmet of salvation, and the sword of the Spirit, which is the word of God." (Ephesians 6:17 ESV)

FURTHER THOUGHTS

- What is your relationship with Scripture/the Bible?
- Do you struggle with reading and understanding it?
- Do you need tools to help you study?
- Do you need accountability to make the time for it?

GOING OLD SCHOOL

*"The priest is to go outside the camp and examine them.
If they have been healed of their defiling skin disease, the
priest shall order that two live clean birds and some cedar
wood, scarlet yarn and hyssop be brought for the person
to be cleansed." (Leviticus 14:3–4 NIV)*

'VE ALWAYS FOUND it intriguing and even telling that
in the Old Testament, the priests were the ones who handled medical issues. How many pastors do you know who
also went to medical school?

It's not that the priests practiced medicine or were what
we might label as apothecaries, but there were instructions in
the Law on how to handle the birthing of a child, burns, or
even boils (see Leviticus 12–14). When God spoke protocols
for these things, He gave them to Aaron and Moses. These
guys weren't doctors, but were leaders, priests, and prophets.

From the beginning, God knew what He was doing, and
He designed us so that the spiritual is connected to the physical. This doesn't mean to ditch your doctor, but you do need
to understand that there is a deep element to wellness that a
pill cannot reach. Medicine and medical practice are critical,
but we can't eliminate the spiritual component.

All throughout the Bible we see healing from the Old Testament to the New. Jesus had a profound impact in healing that doesn't get a lot of credit in the medical world. John testified that Jesus did so many things that the world couldn't contain the books if they were recorded (John 21:25). That is a medical breakthrough!

That claim by John is not just some half-hearted thought included in the last part of the Gospel. This is a glimpse of what the power of Christ can do in our lives to this day. But on this journey of mental wellness, you may need to reconsider what you think Jesus can do in you and for you.

> "If I can?" Jesus asked. "Anything is possible
> if you have faith." (Mark 9:23 TLB)

FURTHER THOUGHTS

- Do you realize the connection between the physical and the spiritual? If not, why?
- Do you believe that God can do anything in your own life? Where is the limit and why?

LET'S GET SPIRITUAL, SPIRITUAL . . .

"It is true that I am an ordinary, weak human being, but I
don't use human plans and methods to win my battles.
I use God's mighty weapons, not those made by men,
to knock down the devil's strongholds."
(2 Corinthians 10:3–4 TLB)

YES, TODAY'S TITLE is a lame play on the old Olivia Newton John song. It's cheesy, but you have to give me points for trying. Besides, it's kinda catchy, right?

When we talk about mental and emotional wellness, we are talking about a battle on the inside, about the inward parts of us. Those inward parts of us are our thoughts and emotions. And while thoughts and emotions entail a lot, there's more to it.

Biblically, you never see verses about the brain. The Bible talks about the mind instead. That's because the mind is the spiritual equal to the brain. The mind is connected to the brain. (Dr. Caroline Leaf is a great resource on this.)

In the same fashion, the soul and the heart (the seat of your affections) are the spiritual equal to the heart (the organ in your chest). The physical parts of the body have a spiritual counterpart connected to them. This concept is far from simple to fully unpack.

Keep this in mind when discussing the mental and emotional change you want in your life. This change is an inward, spiritual work as well as an outward, physical work.

For me, some things took a couple years to change. Other issues took decades. With some things, I'm still under construction. I don't say that to discourage you, but to let you know that you have a comrade-in-arms who has stuck in there to see breakthroughs and miracles—and that there is hope for those of us who are thick-headed!

So get a long-haul mentality about this wellness journey and be patient. As a mentor often says, "Persistence is often the greatest revenge on hell." So persist is exactly what we must do.

> *"But I tell you this—though he won't do it for friendship's sake, if you keep knocking long enough, he will get up and give you whatever you need because of your shameless persistence." (Luke 11:8 NLT)*

FURTHER THOUGHTS

- Are you a persistent person or do you struggle with defeat?
- Is there anything you've given up on changing in you? What is it?

I STAND CORRECTED

"Those whom I [dearly and tenderly] love, I rebuke and discipline [showing them their faults and instructing them]; so be enthusiastic and repent [change your inner self—your old way of thinking, your sinful behavior—seek God's will]."
(Revelation 3:19 AMP)

IT TOOK ME a very long time to become the type of person who could receive correction. I couldn't handle it from others and I certainly couldn't handle it from God. I wrestled with Him for years before I truly saw change in my life. I fought tooth and nail with Him on everything because I missed a critical part of my walk with God—His love for me.

I had stories about Him showing me His love. I even had them journaled and read them over and over again. I had memorized verses about His love. But still no revelation. What I lacked in love, I made up for with a giant chip on my shoulder.

Not to give myself an excuse, but that giant chip was there for good reason. It was the evidence of the mental and emotional struggles I had since early childhood—struggles that almost took me out several times.

When I finally got the revelation of the love of God, it changed me . . . literally. You see, people who can't be corrected don't understand love. Those who don't understand love will be at a stalemate with God until they do.

The reason correction and discipline are vital in love is because we have to recognize the things in us that obstruct or destroy love (which is God—see 1 John 4:8). A person who is well-loved can be corrected in almost anything because they understand the motive behind the correction.

Ridding toxic patterns. Overcoming fears and insecurities. Changing cycles of generational issues. Breaking mindsets. Finding freedom from habits. These all stem from a healthy center of love.

I'm not saying it's easy to hear or receive correction (or that it ever will be), but you will no longer dig in your heels or dispute the truth. It is still a process. Learning about the love of God is not a one-time thing, but rather a life-long journey. That ol' chip is hard to kill off when it was a part of your life for so long.

Take an honest look at yourself. Have you been hitting a wall with breakthrough? If yes, ask this—can you be confronted? If no, then you most likely have an issue of love on your hands. And while you can't self-manufacture that change, your first step is to pray for God to change that.

"And may you have the power to understand, as all God's
people should, how wide, how long, how high, and how
deep his love is. May you experience the love of Christ,
though it is too great to understand fully. Then you will be

made complete with all the fullness of life and power that
comes from God." (Ephesians 3:18–19 NLT)

FURTHER THOUGHTS

- Revisit the questions in the last paragraph. Is there room for improvement?

A LIE ABOUT THE TRUTH

"If you love Me, keep My commandments. And I will pray
the Father, and He will give you another Helper, that He
may abide with you forever— the Spirit of truth, whom
the world cannot receive, because it neither sees Him nor
knows Him; but you know Him, for He dwells with you
and will be in you." (John 14:15–17 NKJV)

W E'VE ALREADY UNCOVERED that the battle for continual improvement in mental and emotional wellness is one that is deeply connected to our spiritual nature. Besides salvation and Scripture, the biggest asset for this journey is the Holy Spirit. You cannot overestimate how important the Holy Spirit is for you in every aspect of life.

Many people have misconceptions about the Holy Spirit. Having misconceptions about the Holy Spirit could possibly be a grave mistake, so it's imperative not to gloss over this or tune it out. With mental issues impacting inside the Church worldwide, general knowledge just won't cut it.

The average, unchurched Joe thinks all churches are either boring and dry as a bone, or completely crazy—running around, handling snakes, and speaking in tongues (that was my impression anyways). Anything "spiritual" was weird and people usually found it to be hokey because they suddenly become unspiritual as soon as the church service ends. Now, I'm not taking shots at any denomination here. I am pointing out that perspectives like this are not balanced or truthful.

One of the titles Jesus gave the Holy Spirit was the "Spirit of truth," and it's not a surprise to me that there are so many misunderstandings or false perceptions about Him. Coincidence? Nah, it's a ploy of the devil, for he is the father of lies (John 8:44).

Knowing this tactic of the devil to shroud the Holy Spirit with lies and misunderstandings is foundational. This knowledge will remove any estrangement towards the Holy Spirit, and we will welcome Him into our hearts with open arms. The more we utilize and welcome the Holy Spirit, the more freedom we will experience.

At this point, stop and pray. Speak directly to the Holy Spirit. A powerful and simple prayer you can start with is by asking to know about Him, the Spirit of truth.

> *"In the same way the Spirit [comes to us and] helps us in our weakness. We do not know what prayer to offer or how to offer it as we should, but the Spirit Himself [knows our need and at the right time] intercedes on our behalf with sighs and groanings too deep for words."*
> *(Romans 8:26 AMP)*

FURTHER THOUGHTS

- What is your understanding of and relationship with the Holy Spirit?

- Where can you improve your relationship with the Holy Spirit?

MORE THAN A
HELPING

*"I have told you these things while I am still with you. But
the Helper (Comforter, Advocate, Intercessor—Counselor,
Strengthener, Standby), the Holy Spirit, whom the Father
will send in My name [in My place, to represent Me and act
on My behalf], He will teach you all things. And He
will help you remember everything that I have told you."*
(John 14:25–26 AMP)

HEARING SOMEONE'S NAME can either bring a
smile to your face or make you cringe. However, in
the Bible, names had more than a reputation; they
had prophetic meaning. Today we see another name that
Jesus gave the Holy Spirit.

Depending on what translation you're reading, you might
see Advocate, Helper, or even Comforter. The name in Greek
indicates one that was "called to one's aid."

While that's just putting it simply, that understanding is
enough to get the big picture. The Holy Spirit's job and role is
to come alongside us to help, comfort, and advocate on our
behalf. He is not only *a* helper, but *the* Helper.

Just like medicine, the Holy Spirit works on the inside of us. His duty is to be alongside us. Contrary to popular belief, you don't get "possessed by the Holy Ghost" and lose all control. This is a partnership.

The help and comfort that the Holy Spirit gives is crucial for mental and emotional wellness. Often, we struggle with feeling alone and overwhelmed, and when we do, we can start spiraling or making regrettable decisions that we can't undo. Instead, we have another option—the best option.

In times of depression, pray for the tangible comfort of the Holy Spirit. Believe that you are not alone, despite your feelings, and that the Holy Spirit is with you. This Helper isn't simply obligated to help, He wants to because He loves you.

The Holy Spirit does so much that it is hard to describe it all in mere words. The key to our improvement and wellness is to partner with Him daily. Building upon our relationship with the Holy Spirit is essential, but don't get overwhelmed. Just take it little by little and let the Comforter, Helper, and Advocate do just that in your life.

> "But when the truth-giving Spirit comes, he will unveil the reality of every truth within you. He won't speak his own message, but only what he hears from the Father, and he will reveal prophetically to you what is to come."
> (John 16:13 TPT)

FURTHER THOUGHTS
- What are the areas that you need the Holy Spirit's help and partnership?

- How can you partner with the Holy Spirit to improve these areas?

YOU HAVE MORE INFLUENCE THAN YOU THINK

"For the mind-set of the flesh is death, but the mind-set controlled by the Spirit finds life and peace."
(Romans 8:6 TPT)

THE AVERAGE PERSON thinks thousands of thoughts per day. Yes, thousands. Now, let me ask you this—how many of those thoughts do you think are positive?

The thoughts that you think are the most influential part of your life. Yes, you are your biggest influence. Not your spouse, boss, or parent. That seems like a lot of responsibility, right?

What you think will impact your health in either a negative or positive way. You can't ruminate with toxic self-talk and expect to get a positive impact. However, the massive overhaul required to do a 180° change in our thought life can seem daunting, if not impossible.

Just a few verses before today's verse, the Apostle Paul

says there is no condemnation for those in Christ. I love this, because I am my own biggest critic. The amount of judgmental, condemning thoughts I think is absurd. I've been doing it for years and only recently have I been catching on to how toxic I can be to myself.

You'll never totally get rid of negative or toxic thoughts, but you can catch on to them and replace them. If it takes one little mustard seed of faith to move a mountain, then use one small thought to start changing your life. One moment, one thought at a time, you'll see a difference. With the help of the Holy Spirit, you absolutely can change your thinking.

Here is the first little step to take: be intentional today to contemplate one thought, idea, or verse. Just one. Set an alarm to remind yourself of it or write it several places to get your attention. Then once that settles in for a week or two, use a different verse or thought.

> *"He told them, 'It was because of your lack of faith. I promise you, if you have faith inside of you no bigger than the size of a small mustard seed, you can say to this mountain, "Move away from here and go over there," and you will see it move! There is nothing you couldn't do!"'*
> (Matthew 17:20 TPT)

FURTHER THOUGHTS
- Do you recognize certain recurring toxic thoughts?
- What Scripture can you use to replace those toxic thoughts?

OUT OF OPTIONS

*"I call heaven and earth to witness against you that today
I have set before you life or death, blessing or curse. Oh,
that you would choose life; that you and your children
might live!" (Deuteronomy 30:19 TLB)*

I F YOU THINK that just because you go to church or that you are a person of faith that you are exempt from mental illness, you're deceived. I don't mean that to be harsh, but you can't afford to be mistaken. Pastors and people in ministry commit suicide. It's heartbreaking, but it happens.

If you're a born-again Christian, then it's likely that the battle for you is even harder. The devil hates anything God loves, so you and I are fair game. Since the battle is hard, we have to understand what's really going on in the spiritual realm and how it impacts our thoughts, all the way down to our physical health.

One of the biggest factors in my own breakthrough and life change boils down to one factor—I made up my mind that quitting is never an option. That's right. No matter how hard things were or how fed up I was, quitting (by means of suicide or otherwise) is out of the question.

It didn't mean that I didn't want to or that such thoughts

never came when things were at their worst. It just means that I chose life every time. I chose to fight. I chose to remain, no matter how badly I faced failure and discouragement. It didn't matter how terrible things were or how ugly my life was; I refused to quit.

Life is going to get ugly because we live in a time of waiting for the return of Christ. Until that happens, the enemy will try to cause chaos in and around us. We must anchor ourselves in Christ.

Failures will happen. Regrets will haunt you. People will quit on you. You will quit on you. But God will never quit on you. He will always be on the inside fighting for you, believing the best for you because He has better for you. So make up your mind here and now—**quitting isn't an option**.

> *"You need to keep on patiently doing God's will if you want him to do for you all that he has promised."*
> (Hebrews 10:36 TLB)

FURTHER THOUGHTS

- Are suicidal thoughts a struggle for you? If so, tell someone. Get accountability and help. Call the Suicide and Crisis Lifeline by dialing 988. (And if you have no one else, tell me.)

IT'S TIME FOR A COMEBACK

*"The godly may trip seven times, but they will get up
again. But one disaster is enough to overthrow the wicked."
(Proverbs 24:16 NLT)*

NOW THAT WE'VE determined that quitting isn't
an option, we need to address how to handle failure.
Handling failure is essential to your mental/emotional wellness and its impact on your success.

Just because we are in Christ doesn't mean we are perfect.
The verse states that the righteous fall seven times and get
back up. Yep, the righteous fall.

Like it or not, everyone will fall. Righteous or not, we
all fail. It's what you do after you fail that will make all the
difference. The wicked fall and never bounce back. But the
righteous make a comeback. As author and Bible teacher
Beth Moore says, "In order to have a comeback, you have to
come back."

I'm not making light of failure, but I am simplifying it. I
have gone through devastating failure and have had to find
my way through it when I thought good could never come

of it. But that is what God can do. He can take the absolute worst and make it beautiful. There's nothing too hard for Him (Jer. 32:27).

Paul instructed us to take who we are and become more and more like Jesus until we reflect Him (2 Cor. 3:18). That includes our failures. The worst of me that I battled with the most is no longer the "worst of me" because I failed and got back up enough times and God kept teaching me and giving me grace. Trial and error with God eventually transformed me.

There were some things that I easily dropped when God showed me they were wrong according to Scripture. Other things took several years or even decades to slowly break free from, *but* I *did* break free from them. Since God has no favorites, you can too.

It may take hours in Scripture and prayer. It may take thousands of failures, but you *can* get back up, because Jesus did! The power that helped Him overcome death, hell, and the grave is the exact same power that lives in you and me.

So shake the dust off. Put a bandage on the scrapes. Let go of the embarrassment of falling yet again, and get back up!

"But if the Spirit of Him who raised Jesus from the dead
dwells in you, He who raised Christ from the dead will also
give life to your mortal bodies through His Spirit
who dwells in you." (Romans 8:11 NKJV)

FURTHER THOUGHTS
- Do you struggle with the idea of perfection? Why or why not?
- How do you handle failure? In a toxic or healthy way?

DETOX

"Get rid of all bitterness . . ." (Ephesians 4:32 NLT)

SOMETIMES A GOOD ol' detox is necessary to jumpstart a journey to health and wellness. While I'm not a huge advocate of doing them physically, I do love to do a spiritual one. Today can mark the beginning of yours.

Unforgiveness is often one of the largest areas of toxicity and sickness in a Christian. It is pointless to ask Christ for forgiveness for our sins and shortcomings but deny it to others. Yet that's exactly what we do if we do not forgive. We keep holding this unforgiveness towards people, waiting to hear an apology from them while our hearts become more and more hardened and sick.

Jesus said that our forgiveness hinges on whether we forgive others (Matt. 6:14). He modeled forgiving others in the Lord's Prayer. He was still forgiving folks in His final moments leading up to His death on the cross (Luke 23:34).

Forgiveness isn't just *recommended* for our soul's well-being, it is *necessary*. Whatever a person did to you, no matter how much it hurts, let it go in the hands of God. Release it to Him to free yourself from the burden of revenge.

He knows how to handle people and judge them without causing further damage. Trust Him to deal with others because *your* forgiveness is at stake.

Ask God to search your heart to reveal *all* unforgiveness. If you need to, make a list and ask Him to help you let them and the offenses go. It's time to detox.

"But if you refuse to forgive others, your Father will not forgive your sins." (Matthew 6:15 NLT)

FURTHER THOUGHTS

- Take a moment to pray and ask God if you hold any hidden unforgiveness. If anyone comes to mind, pray and ask God to help you let go of the offense.

WE AIN'T DONE

"For we also have received the good news just as they did;
but the message they heard did not benefit them, since they
were not united with those who heard it in faith."
(Hebrews 4:2 CSB)

HOW MANY TIMES have you listened to sermons or heard the Gospel preached and it had no impact on you? Or maybe it impacted the person next to you, but not you? When this happens time and time again, we lose faith and hope in the power of God and we seek out other things to satisfy us or meet our needs. We have to frequently ask ourselves where we rest our faith. The writer of Hebrews implies that the message or Gospel had no impact because it wasn't coupled with faith.

Everyone has faith or belief in something. But it's what you join your faith to that matters. As Christians, our faith in anything other than the message of Jesus is actually wrong. Anything but Christ or even anything added to Christ isn't pure faith.

False faith can be quite an issue. It renders you powerless and leads you down pathways of deceit. Here are examples of false faith:

- Do you believe in magic?
- How about making wishes?
- Horoscopes?
- Energy crystals?
- Water witching or dowsing?
- Luck?
- Psychics and/or mediums?

Those things directly oppose Jesus, no matter how innocent you make them out to be.

When I first started going to church, I practiced tarot card reading. I dabbled in other stuff too, but tarot cards were something I really enjoyed. I never used them in a dark sense, so I thought it was alright. Then I realized that Scripture speaks against all forms of divination, witchcraft, or spiritism. I immediately stopped and repented.

I know the arguments and how innocent it can appear, but there is deception in these practices right down to the smallest ways. It completely leads your faith astray from the *only* one who knows your destiny and future. Any deceit we believe will eventually lead us away from God and into more confusion and problems.

Take a moment and check what you believe in. This is another form of detox we need to do. Assess where you place your faith and direct it to good and healthy things, such as the church, the Bible, and the Holy Spirit. Ask God to show you things that have displaced your belief in Christ alone. Perhaps the reason church or the Bible seems so powerless is because you have diluted your faith. Resting in the Good News of Christ alone is power enough.

"*Now the practices of the sinful nature are clearly evident: they are sexual immorality, impurity, sensuality (total irresponsibility, lack of self-control), idolatry, sorcery, hostility, strife, jealousy, fits of anger, disputes, dissensions, factions [that promote heresies], envy, drunkenness, riotous behavior, and other things like these. I warn you beforehand, just as I did previously, that those who practice such things will not inherit the kingdom of God.*"
(Galatians 5:19–21 AMP)

FURTHER THOUGHTS

- What have you sought outside of God that has impacted your faith?
- Are there items or things you need to get rid of in order set things right (i.e., tarot cards or charms)?

TIME HEALS ALL
WOUNDS (?)

*"Confess and acknowledge how you have offended one
another and then pray for one another to be instantly
healed, for tremendous power is released through the
passionate, heartfelt prayer of a godly believer!"*
(James 5:16 TPT)

CTUALLY, NO, TIME doesn't heal all wounds.
Time helps you forget or lets your emotions cool
down, but if you don't deal with your fears and hurts,
it will impact every part of you and you'll go to the grave with
those wounds.

You know what does heal? Confession.

We already talked about forgiveness being a key factor in
cleansing our hearts before God, but confession is also vital.
It seems to be a lost practice outside of some denominations.
Maybe it's because we misunderstand its purpose.

It's not about God holding the light over us like an investigator, drilling us as suspects, ready to pounce on us with
accusations. That doesn't even line up with the character of
God revealed in Scripture. Instead, God designed confession

to heal. Interestingly enough, the Greek word James used for "healing" mainly referred to physical healing (although spiritual healing is encompassed).

Let that sink in. When was the last time you confessed sin? It is either time you did it again, or time to start incorporating it in your life.

Ask God to give you a trustworthy, safe friend to confess your junk to. Don't just confess cheating on your diet either. Dig deep. Talk about your insecurities, jealousy, or the shame you may struggle with.

Don't take confession flippantly, but let God lead you as you ask Him to reveal areas that need healing. The depth of your healing is equivalent to how deep you let God take you. If you don't have another person to confess to, you can still confess to Jesus. He's the one who sticks closer than a brother anyways.

"But if we freely admit our sins when his light uncovers them, he will be faithful to forgive us every time. God is just to forgive us our sins because of Christ, and he will continue to cleanse us from all unrighteousness." (1 John 1:9 TPT)

FURTHER THOUGHTS

- Evaluate your level of honesty with God. Do you really let Him inspect your heart? If not, what holds you back?
- Is there anything you need to confess in prayer? If so, take some time to do it.

WHAT'S THE BIG IDEA?

"We are destroying sophisticated arguments and every
exalted and proud thing that sets itself up against the
[true] knowledge of God, and we are taking every thought
and purpose captive to the obedience of Christ . . ."
(2 Corinthians 10:5 AMP)

PRAYED AND PRAYED and prayed for a miracle in my life. I didn't get it. Some of my struggles I had been battling for my entire life. Why wasn't God changing this? I had seen Him answer other people's prayers; why not mine?

Twenty years later, I can tell you that He had another plan for me. I had a lot of hatred towards God. A lot of complaints. A lot of doing it my own way, failing, and coming back at Him with hurt and anger. And then I learned the truth.

My freedom hinged on unlearning what I had believed and been taught my entire life and relearning how to think according to the Bible. This is also called breaking a stronghold. Discovering one lie at a time, replacing it with truth from Scripture, and repeating that process has changed my life over time.

You see, the devil is a liar. Anything that he can get us to believe and hide in apart from God creates negative strong-

34

holds. Negative strongholds keep us chained up in destructive cycles, even after accepting Christ as Savior. But there is another option.

Not all strongholds are bad. God can be our stronghold. His presence and promises can be the safe place for us to run to, mentally and emotionally.

This isn't easy. I don't want you to misunderstand me. Breaking a stronghold usually doesn't happen in a moment (it can, but for me it never did). But never underestimate how relentless persistence can pay off over time.

Breaking a stronghold usually starts with becoming aware of it. Then little by little, every time a feeling brings a contrary thought, refute it with a verse of truth. Over time, things snowball and change. Habits change and no longer hold power over you.

If you've never heard of or done this before, start with prayer. Ask God to show you where these strongholds are in your life. Look for places you get defensive; usually that shows you where a lie is hiding.

I'll be praying for you. I'm excited that freedom is on the brink. Keep moving forward, no matter how long it takes!

> *"The Lord is my fort where I can enter and be safe; no one can follow me in and slay me. He is a rugged mountain where I hide; he is my Savior, a rock where none can reach me, and a tower of safety. He is my shield. He is like the strong horn of a mighty fighting bull." (Psalm 18:2 TLB)*

FURTHER THOUGHTS
- Are you aware of obvious strongholds in your life?

- What lie are you believing that you can replace with the truth of Scripture?

FROM THE INSIDE OUT

"Stop imitating the ideals and opinions of the culture
around you, but be inwardly transformed by the Holy Spirit
through a total reformation of how you think."
(Romans 12:2a TPT)

YESTERDAY WE TALKED about strongholds. Today we'll expand on that idea with transformation.

Change is inevitable. You don't really have a choice about it either. Whether it's your body aging, the seasons bringing different weather, or even just life events turning the tide—change happens. We may not have much control over what happens to us, but we can control how we respond to it.

Paul references the idea of *conforming* in Romans 12. Conforming is a process that copies other things or customs. It is merely a rearranging of things on the outside of your life that gives a false notion of change. It takes inspiration from an outside environment and models after it. This is what Paul says *not* to do.

The second choice Paul mentions is *transformation*. This process is where we get our term "metamorphosis" in English—a caterpillar changing into a butterfly. It doesn't just impact one part of a thing, but the whole of it, and it works from the inside out.

Those two choices are our options. What you decide will dictate how you change. However, the better choice is transformation. Transformation is the result of the Holy Spirit and Scripture changing how we think.

Transformation directly impacts and creates new life. The old thoughts, that created old emotions, that created old behaviors, that created your old self is to be interjected with a renewal of thoughts from Scripture. This will impact you by replacing that old process with better thoughts to create breakthroughs until the whole of you is changed from the inside out.

Like the butterfly, it may start out ugly and haggard, but it will eventually change into something beautiful and completely different. Have patience; the process is well worth it.

"Therefore if anyone is in Christ [that is, grafted in, joined to Him by faith in Him as Savior], he is a new creature [reborn and renewed by the Holy Spirit]; the old things [the previous moral and spiritual condition] have passed away. Behold, new things have come [because spiritual awakening brings a new life]." (2 Corinthians 5:17 AMP)

FURTHER THOUGHTS

- What things or areas do you want transformed in you (not just edited, but a complete change)?

THE BEST IS
YET TO COME

*"Then you will learn from your own experience how his
ways will really satisfy you." (Romans 12:2b TLB)*

LOOK YA'LL, TRANSFORMATION ain't no joke.
Paul's command of transformation doesn't just happen
overnight with little trial and error. I didn't have a
"Damascus Road experience" that completely changed the
trajectory of my life in a matter of days. Transformation has
taken the better part of twenty years for me, and I'm still
under construction. But this command from Romans isn't
to punish us or because God is some weird power-tripping
dictator. There's a method to the madness.

Paul instructs us to renew our mind so that we will know
God's will for us. The "good, pleasing, and perfect" will that
Paul talks about is not just from God's perspective, but from
what He knows will be "good, pleasing, and perfect" in your
perspective also. Read that again.

That's not just some gimmick. It's not too good to be true.
Yes, transformation is a process (albeit grueling at times), but
it's *for* us. It's for us to know what's best in our life.

You have a choice though. You can stick to the same ol' diet that everyone else is munching on every day. Anxiety. Toxicity. Out of control emotions and thinking. Or you can surrender your will to get to know His. It will require all of you, but isn't the best worth that?

> *"Look at the birds! They don't worry about what to eat—*
> *they don't need to sow or reap or store up food—for your*
> *heavenly Father feeds them. And you are far more valuable*
> *to him than they are." (Matthew 6:26 TLB)*

FURTHER THOUGHTS

- Deep down in your bones, do you trust that God has your best in mind? Why or why not?
- Where do you need to relinquish control and trust Him?

YOU'RE NOT JUST
HEARING THINGS

"The sheep that are My own hear My voice and listen to Me;
I know them, and they follow Me." (John 10:27 AMP)

EOPLE TALK ABOUT how crazy people hear voices.
I don't believe they are necessarily crazy. Everyone
hears voices. Now before you think I'm freaky, hang on
tight as I elaborate.

Every person has two voices they always hear: their own
or an evil spirit's. As a Christian, there are three voices we
hear in our thoughts—ours, a spirit's, and God's. Don't let
this knowledge freak you out. We need to understand this to
navigate transforming our thought life.

The Bible is the *logos* of God (Greek meaning "logic"). So
we essentially have God's thinking or how God thinks for us
to sift through and apply to our lives. Also, Scripture specifically states that we have the mind of Christ by the Holy Spirit
(1 Cor. 2:16). These two factors are huge.

The more we access the mind of Christ spiritually and
the more we align our thinking to agree with the promises
of God (a.k.a. the Bible), the more we can decipher which

thoughts we should listen to and which to avoid. Your own thoughts may be good, but they are not the best (only God knows what's best for us). And as for an evil spirit's thoughts, we know we don't want that junk, because it will lead us further from God and deeper into cycles of addictions, strongholds, irrational and unhealthy fears, and the like.

Transforming our thoughts will show us God's best for us. This is God's desire for our life as we learn to listen to the right thoughts. So no, you're not crazy, but the thoughts you give in to will determine the direction of your life.

"And we have received God's Spirit (not the world's spirit), so we can know the wonderful things God has freely given us."
(1 Corinthians 2:12 NLT)

FURTHER THOUGHTS

- What is the overall tone of your thought life? Positive? Negative? Condemning?
- Which recurring thoughts need to be addressed with the logic of Scripture?

DON'T GO THERE

"An unfriendly person isolates himself and seems to care only about his own issues. For his contempt of sound judgment makes him a recluse." (Proverbs 18:1 TPT)

B Y "THERE," I mean isolation. I've seen this so many times that I lost count. I've done it myself and seen many people fall off the wagon, not realizing what they are doing. While you don't have to struggle with mental and emotional issues to do this, it seems to be a trap for those who do.

Listen closely—stop pulling away from people. Stop falling out of contact from the healthy and accountable relationships in your life. Stop binging on TV and self-medicating. It's costing you more than you realize.

"I just need some me time." "I just need some time to recover and find myself." I know that argument because I've used it myself. There is *some* truth to those statements. However, how you go about doing it is important. We all know that Jesus would go and be away from people to connect with God and pray.

What you pull away *from* and go *to* in your "me time" is telling. The Bible calls isolation flat-out selfish. All selfishness is toxic and unhealthy. Yep, that can be offensive to how we think, but unless you handle correction well, you'll keep repeating cycles of selfish behavior that lead you further away from God.

The truth is that we thrive in community. We are designed to connect. In fact, studies show that healing increases over 60% when done in community. As the Church, we are all a part of something bigger than ourselves. The next time you're tempted to isolate (which will happen since selfishness is a natural go-to for the flesh), reach out to God or a friend instead of pulling away. Refuse to isolate mentally and physically.

Go take a bath and pray. Or go walk and pray. It may not be what you want, but it's what you need. It makes a world of difference, mentally and emotionally, how we handle these moments.

> *"So you must remain in life-union with me, for I remain in life-union with you. For as a branch severed from the vine will not bear fruit, so your life will be fruitless unless you live your life intimately joined to mine." (John 15:4 TPT)*

FURTHER THOUGHTS

- Do you struggle with isolating yourself? Why?
- Do you see the lie in isolation?
- What can you do instead the next time you want to push away from God and others?

UNPOPULAR OPINION

"For where jealousy and selfish ambition exist, there is disorder [unrest, rebellion] and every evil thing and morally degrading practice." (James 3:16 AMP)

ONE OF THE biggest secrets in the battle for mental health is that in order to conquer this demon you must focus on something other than yourself and your issues. I don't say this to offend you, but because it is important for your freedom.

Before you shut me down with a rebuttal, I understand that I don't know your specific problems, but think about it. If you're constantly thinking about your own anxiety, fears, or needs, then what are your thoughts centered on? You. The "I'ma do me" or "I need to go find myself" or "this doesn't serve me" attitude of our culture is one of the biggest deceptions from the devil, and I'm not being overly spiritual.

The biggest breakthroughs that have impacted my life were when I served a greater purpose than myself. Missions, women's ministry, and the Momentum Monday Devotional email are all things that God used to change my life because they forced me to think about others.

Contrary to popular opinion and thought in our culture,

your life isn't about pleasing you. It's actually about pleasing God. He loves it when we serve and put others over ourselves.

You thrive when you meet the needs of or help others. So when you feel at your lowest (and those moments will always come), think of a way to combat that. Go serve somewhere. Check in on a friend. Text a friend and encourage them.

We were made for something bigger than ourselves. Even Jesus, the man who impacted history the most, said that His purpose wasn't to be served but to serve (Matt. 20:28). Besides, what do you have to lose by recentering your life around something other than your anxiety?

> *"Do nothing from selfishness or empty conceit [through factional motives, or strife], but with [an attitude of] humility [being neither arrogant nor self-righteous], regard others as more important than yourselves. Do not merely look out for your own personal interests, but also for the interests of others. Have this same attitude in yourselves which was in Christ Jesus [look to Him as your example in selfless humility] . . ." (Philippians 2:3–5 AMP)*

FURTHER THOUGHTS

- What self-focused issues can you see that need to be more focused on God and/or others?

THIS TOO SHALL PASS

"The steadfast love of the LORD never ceases; his mercies never come to an end; they are new every morning; great is your faithfulness." (Lamentations 3:22–23 ESV)

SN'T IT INTRIGUING that our bad days and bad seasons seem like they will never end? Isn't it odd that we seem to lose all hope in the middle of those moments? Or that good times seem so fleeting and bad ones drag on and on?

One of the best things I've learned to do in the midst of hopeless moments is to remember that it's just a moment. When I'm mentally, physically, or emotionally drained, I'll find myself being very negative, thinking some of my worst thoughts because my emotions are in the driver's seat. But as quick as that thought comes, I remind myself not to take that thought seriously and to move on. Tomorrow or next week will be better.

The reason I believe and rely on that thought is because it's true. God's mercies for us are new every morning. We're not promised only good days and good experiences in life, but we are promised mercy, love, and grace. We're promised the help of the Holy Spirit.

Regardless of how you're feeling or how long you've felt it, start believing in the mercy of God for you. Don't hang on to negative thoughts; let them go as quickly as they come. Trust that better days are ahead. Because of Jesus, they are!

"Lord, be gracious to us! We wait for You. Be our strength every morning and our salvation in time of trouble."
(Isaiah 33:2 CSB)

FURTHER THOUGHTS

- Looking back over tough times, do you see God's mercy in those seasons? Why or why not?
- In what ways can you better handle bad days?

A GRASSHOPPER'S FRAME OF MIND

"There we saw the Nephilim (the sons of Anak are part of
the Nephilim); and we were like grasshoppers in our own
sight, and so we were in their sight." (Numbers 13:33 AMP)

THIS CHAPTER TEACHES a very valuable lesson. God had given the Israelites the land of Canaan, but at the time, giants roamed the land. Moses sent a team of people from each tribe of Israel to scout the land and come back with a report.

Out of the twelve who went to spy out the land, only two had faith to want to go take possession. The other ten came back with a fearful report. Granted, any human would be afraid of giants, but the ten had forgotten something in the face of giants: the size of their God and what He had promised.

The land was rightfully theirs. God had already given them a promise that they would possess it. Anything that God promises, He will enable. But because they saw themselves as puny and weak, which distracted them from the power of God, they portrayed themselves to others as puny and weak.

You are created in the image of God. A skewed perspective of yourself means you have a skewed vision of God. It's like looking at yourself in a clown mirror. The reflection is there, but it's distorted.

You can't afford to lose sight of the power of your Creator. Our Promised Land requires us to conquer giants, not in our own confidence, but God's. Losing sight of Him makes us shoulder problems on our own.

What you focus on, you magnify. Keep God's promises on your mind. Keep the size and power of God on your mind. You are not a grasshopper, but a child of God.

"So God created human beings in his own image. In the image of God he created them; male and female he created them." (Genesis 1:27 NLT)

FURTHER THOUGHTS

- Looking at the giants facing you in your life, how big do you make God in comparison to them?
- Are there any promises that God has given you that you have forgotten about? If so, what are they?

GETTING YOUR
HOPES UP

*"When hope's dream seems to drag on and on, the delay can
be depressing. But when at last your dream comes true, life's
sweetness will satisfy your soul." (Proverbs 13:12 TPT)*

A SURE-FIRE WAY TO never get disappointed is to never get your hopes up. Don't have any expectations and you won't have any disappointments. Right? I operated like this for a long time until I came to a deep realization.

The ordeals of your life hinge on how you steward your heart (Prov. 4:23). Every single issue that you have doesn't point back to your parents and how they raised you (though that does have some influence) or how much money you have (or don't have). Everything points to how you govern your heart.

Where do you put your hope? Who do you hope in? What is at the foundation of all you hope for? Those answers are crucial to understanding why your soul struggles with depression, anxiety, or tension.

When we rest our hope in a person, goal, or situation and

it doesn't pull through, the heart breaks and becomes bitter. Hence, the depression the verse references.

There is nothing wrong with wanting things surrounding a person, goal, or situation, but when we do this without the prayerful consent of Jesus, we could be setting ourselves up for heartbreak.

For years, I prayed for dreams and situations to come to pass and I became more and more angry at God at every passing season that it didn't happen. I blamed Him for my toxic, broken heart. But not once did I ever stop to consider if these ideas I prayed for were what God thought was best for me. Nor did I realize that resting my hope on anything outside of God was an opportunity for heartbreak.

Don't stop hoping just because you don't want to be let down again. Instead, adjust your approach. Stop and pray to ask God what He wants for you. His hope never disappoints us.

> *"And patient endurance will refine our character, and proven character leads us back to hope. And this hope is not a disappointing fantasy, because we can now experience the endless love of God cascading into our hearts through the Holy Spirit who lives in us!"*
> *(Romans 5:4-5 TPT)*

FURTHER THOUGHTS

- Revisit paragraph three and answer the questions.
- Do you need to readjust where your hope is? Why or why not?

ALL WORN OUT

"And he shall speak great words against the most High, and
shall wear out the saints of the most High, and think to
change times and laws: and they shall be given into his
hand until a time and times and the dividing of time."
(Daniel 7:25 KJV)

DANIEL GAVE A boatload of wisdom in one sentence. People who show up anxious or exhausted never show their best self. Breaking a person down slowly is a strategic execution plan of the devil.

Mental health and wellness in general will hinge upon guarding your rest. That means you must learn boundaries. One of the simplest boundaries is the word "no." This is one of the vital reasons why God made a Sabbath and then placed it in the Old Testament's top ten.

For me, I can easily say that the worst seasons of my life all had one huge factor in common—exhaustion. I'm not talking about a few days or weeks, but months (and even some years) of sheer exhaustion. This type of exhaustion was not just a physical thing either, but in every area of my life.

The strategy of the devil will be to try to wear you out, physically, mentally, emotionally, and spiritually. You'll try to balance yourself in one way and he'll try to wear you out in another. Then for his grand finale, he'll attempt to wear you out in every single way.

Don't be dismayed or intimidated, but be equipped. Now that you know one of the tactics, be aware and plan ahead. Knowing "how" is one of the first steps to victory. Make rest a priority and be prepared to utilize your "no" without guilt.

> *"He offers a resting place for me in his luxurious love. His tracks take me to an oasis of peace, the quiet brook of bliss."*
> (Psalm 23:2 TPT)

FURTHER THOUGHTS

- What does rest look like to you?
- Do you keep a Sabbath or place boundaries well?
- How can you improve those boundaries?

AIN'T NOTHING LIKE THE REAL THING, BABY

"For God did not give us a spirit of timidity or cowardice or fear, but [He has given us a spirit] of power and of love and of sound judgment and personal discipline [abilities that result in a calm, well-balanced mind and self-control]."
(2 Timothy 1:7 AMP)

THIS IS THE trifecta of the Christian life. There is more to Christianity than salvation. As vital as salvation is, it is only the beginning of the depth and richness of the Good News of the Gospel.

The advice Paul gave to a young Timothy is not merely head knowledge or inspired revelation. Instead, this is something that Paul learned, and it was part of his own testimony. To testify of the power of the Holy Spirit was a first-hand experience for Paul.

You see, Paul's previous religious zeal was all forced out of the flesh. He was raised knowing the Old Testament by heart, but there was no real power to it. Jesus was a threat to Paul's understanding of God. Up until his Damascus Road experience, he was harassing believers and threatening their lives.

Paul knew the Law and thought he understood the Old Testament, but he had no real understanding of God, Jesus, or the Holy Spirit. You and I must realize the difference between the real and the counterfeit. We often see it in others easily, but it's harder to see it in ourselves.

A legit encounter with Jesus changed Paul's trajectory and marked him for life. He no longer lived trying to control others, but let God deal with him first. With three points, this is where we see law become life.

1. *The Holy Spirit is characterized by power.*
   Fear mimics power by intimidation tactics or false fronts. Paul had been influential by ruling over people with fear, but now he was much more influential with true power from the Holy Spirit.
2. *The Holy Spirit is characterized by love.*
   Love is directly connected to power. Any place that fear resides, love does not. It is fear, not hatred, that is the opposite of love.
3. *The Holy Spirit is characterized by self-control.*
   Power and love are catalysts for sensible behavior via balanced thinking. Trying to control others is a red flag for a lack of control in yourself. Often those who feel powerless and unloved try to generate power by controlling others, but it is a hollow lie.

The job of the Holy Spirit is to lead us out of these types of false living and into truth (John 16:13). It's not behavior modification, but powerful, loving, and sensible living that thrives from the core of the soul. We may be like Paul, with a religious starting point, or may have been saved for decades, but the end goal is to drive out every bit of fear that renders us powerless.

I pray that we would see the false and counterfeit places in ourselves—not for the sake of humility, but to show us where the Holy Spirit needs to work in us most. Then, may God give us the experience to testify to a true impact of the Spirit with power, love, and a sound mind.

> *"And you did not receive the 'spirit of religious duty,' leading you back into the fear of never being good enough. But you have received the 'Spirit of full acceptance,' enfolding you into the family of God. And you will never feel orphaned, for as he rises up within us, our spirits join him in saying the words of tender affection, 'Beloved Father!'"*
> *(Romans 8:15 TPT)*

FURTHER THOUGHTS

- Which of the three (power, love, sound mind) do you struggle with? Why?

BEST PRACTICE

"You will keep the mind that is dependent on You in perfect peace, for it is trusting in You." (Isaiah 26:3 CSB)

I MEMORIZED THIS VERSE years before I knew what it meant. I just knew that it had the words "mind" and "peace" in it, so I just went with it. I knew there was a promise of peace, even if I didn't understand to whom all the pronouns referred.

What I have come to learn is that when my mind is focused on all the chores, to-dos, shoulds, wishes, and worries, I quickly start to see negative emotions flare up. Focusing on me, my, and mine develops a snowball effect that causes an avalanche, and we all know that when avalanches collide with people, the results are never good.

The better thing to do is to focus on God. Whenever our thoughts escape and find their way to Him, the results are usually much different. However, if we need peace (and who doesn't?), there's one more thing to consider.

Peace is a by-product of trust. I can pray all day without trusting Him. All I'm doing is repeating nervous thoughts in list form to Him. But when I pray *and* trust that regardless of the outcome, God has my best interest at heart, then peace abounds.

A person who has resolved all their concerns and has concluded that there is nothing bigger than God, no situation outside of His control, and that underneath it all, God is for their best, will experience perfect peace, as Isaiah says. To get to that conclusion is not easy, but for our sakes, it is best and it is worth it.

> *"Do not be anxious or worried about anything, but in everything [every circumstance and situation] by prayer and petition with thanksgiving, continue to make your [specific] requests known to God." (Philippians 4:6 AMP)*

FURTHER THOUGHTS

- Consider the areas in which you don't have peace. Is your resolve and focus on God? If not, stop and pray (and trust) now.

JUST WHO DO
YOU THINK YOU'RE
TALKING TO?

"Why am I so depressed? Why this turmoil within me?
Put your hope in God, for I will still praise Him,
my Savior and my God." (Psalm 43:5 HCSB)

WE NEED TO take two very important lessons from David in this psalm. First, question your emotions. Second, address your own soul.

Yes, I am telling you to speak to yourself. The first time I heard anybody tell me they did it, I thought they were outside of their ever lovin' mind. But the truth is, your subconscious (the voice in your head) is speaking to you 24/7 and you already speak to yourself. I'm just saying that you need to improve *how* you do it.

Emotions are normal. They are human, but they can be destructive if not checked and/or tamed. As someone once said, "Emotions are like your kids in a car. You don't want them in the driver's seat, but you can't put them in the trunk either."

David spoke to his soul (meaning his mind, will, and emotions) to command his will. Either emotions will drive your will or you can partner with the Holy Spirit to impact your will. This is where the Word of God becomes absolutely imperative. When we choose what God says over what we feel, we are partnering with God's will to empower our will for what is best for us.

"Bless and affectionately praise the Lord, O my soul, And all that is [deep] within me, bless His holy name."
(Psalm 103:1 AMP)

FURTHER THOUGHTS
- How would you classify where your emotions ride in your life? The driver's seat (controlling you)? The passenger seat (your emotions are there, but you do not let them rule you nor do you ignore them)? Or the trunk (pushed to the back and hidden)?
- Why is that?

WHAT MAKES A MAN

"For as he thinks in his heart, so is he."
(Proverbs 23:7a AMPC)

T HE WRITER OF this proverb displays a principle of utmost importance. The quick thought that he incorporates is almost missed if we read too fast. So let's slow down and take in the two vital components derived from this truth.

1. You are not what you do.
   Outward action doesn't comprise who you are. That is a two-way street. Any mistakes that you've made don't define you. Any good you do doesn't either. You can do the right thing with the wrong motive. Your inside content comprises your character.

2. You are what you think.
   If you struggle with anxiety, it's because you think anxious thoughts. If you struggle with anger, it's because you replay past situations that hurt you over and over. Whatever the state of your life, it's due to the quality of your thoughts.

To change that, you don't just change how you think, but you also change what feeds those thoughts. Stop following certain people on the media (social or otherwise). Change which music you listen to. Filter what you watch on TV. Or limit all of those things.

But don't just stop doing something. Replace it. Incorporate other positive, healthy options.

People may judge you by your actions, but that's not the sliding scale that defines our lives. Having a better life and being a better person all boils down to the type of thoughts you think.

> *"For the LORD sees not as man sees; man looks on the*
> *outward appearance, but the LORD looks on the heart."*
> *(1 Samuel 16:7b AMPC)*

FURTHER THOUGHTS
- Where do you need to swap some things out in your life?
- Where do you need to filter things?

THE LIFE YOU'VE ALWAYS WANTED

"Even though I walk through the valley of the shadow of death, I will fear no evil, for you are with me; your rod and your staff, they comfort me." (Psalm 23:4 ESV)

ANY TIME SOMEONE asks a child what they want to be when they grew up, the child never says depressed, angry, broke, or (well, you fill in the blank). Instead, the answer was always some positive reflection in hopes of what they want to be.

The truth is, though, that life is all of it. It's not just the highs, but the lows too. It encompasses everything. We can walk through the valley and fear no evil because of who accompanies us (the Holy Spirit). He is the Comforter in it all.

Nobody wants the lows of life. Death, fear of the unknown, stress, strained relationships, or other negative things leave you deeply discouraged. But that is part of living in today's world.

So often, our reaction is to numb out. Feeling all the lows makes us feel like it will never go away and life will never get any better. However, numbing ourselves with any form of addiction or medication actually keeps us from the abundant life. If we avoid the lows, we will never be able to embrace the highs either. Things like excitement, love, and joy never fully come because we're afraid and trying to prevent the other shoe from dropping (so to speak).

Being a Christian gives us the great privilege of the company of the Holy Spirit. We really should be the most courageous people to walk the earth. Our life doesn't depend on our capacity to handle it all, but on His capacity.

God knows about our unknowns and uncertainties. He knows what we shrink back from and try to avoid. That's why He gave us someone to partner with in the deepest and cruelest parts of life. Lean into the discomfort of the lows with the Holy Spirit. His very job is to comfort. Then hang tight. The promise of abundance will come.

> *"The thief's purpose is to steal and kill and destroy. My purpose is to give them a rich and satisfying life." (John 10:10 NLT)*

FURTHER THOUGHTS

- What are your tendencies in response to stress?
- How can you start leaning more into the Holy Spirit when stress comes?

JUST FOR THE
HEALTH OF IT

"Beloved, I pray that in every way you may
succeed and prosper and be in good health [physically],
just as [I know] your soul prospers [spiritually]."
(3 John 1:2 AMP)

T HE GREEK WORD for *health* in this verse is actually where we get our English word for "hygiene," and for good reason. We define "hygiene" as the proper ways and protocols to maintain good health. And the Greek word for "health" indicates just that: order.

Disfunctions, disorders, diseases, maladies—these are all terms we use when something is not working properly. Someone or something that isn't flowing or working in order has a disconnect or misconnect. To restore health is to restore order (mentally, emotionally, physically, or spiritually).

The depiction of health in Scripture is one of order. God cares about the whole of the person, like the opening of the letter John wrote suggests. To be healthy in body but not in soul (or vice versa) shows a disconnect—a lack of order.

The idea of order has a bigger intent behind it. God is not

a God of order because He is "type A" or anal. It's because there is harmony and fruitfulness when there is unity and order.

One more thought. If God is a God of order, then what do you think the devil is? Yep, his work is characterized by chaos and confusion.

Chaos in our mind. Chaos in our body. Chaos in our emotions. That's tell-tale of the devil's work. Wherever you sense chaos in or around you, that's a clear indication of where we need to pray and let the Holy Spirit work. Any area He shows you, come under the authority and order of the Holy Spirit.

Coming under the authority of God is the pathway to freedom. Further, it's the pathway to order and health in its entirety.

"When Jesus overheard this, he spoke up and said, 'Healthy people don't need to see a doctor, but the sick will go for treatment.'" (Matthew 9:12 TPT)

FURTHER THOUGHTS

- Are there areas where your health (in any manner) is out of order? If so, what are they?
- Stop and ask God to show you where these areas need to change to come under the authority of the Holy Spirit.

FINAL THOUGHTS

"Finally, brothers and sisters, fill your minds with beauty and truth. Meditate on whatever is honorable, whatever is right, whatever is pure, whatever is lovely, whatever is good, whatever is virtuous and praiseworthy."
(Philippians 4:8 VOICE)

YOU'VE PROBABLY READ this verse a lot. If you've been in church for any length of time, you've had to have seen it or heard it preached. But don't lose the value of this verse because of familiarity. There's more depth to this verse than we often realize.

The famous apostle in the New Testament is writing out of gratitude to the church of Philippi. While most of his letters were to address an issue amongst believers, this letter was written to share his love and gratitude for their support. But the best part of his letter was not so much what he said, but where he said it from. Paul was writing from prison.

Prison in the New Testament era was intense. Cable, leisure time, mattresses—none of those conveniences were there. Yet, Paul's circumstances didn't dictate his attitude. What was on the outside didn't control what was happening on the inside. So when Paul tells the Philippian church how to fix their thoughts, we'd be fools not to listen up.

You'd think that the origin of his letter would be enough, but Paul expounds. He doesn't just tell his friends how to think, but tells them that he has known every situation and circumstance, and he has still successfully learned how to be content. Even when he had all the things he wanted, he still had to learn contentment.

Paul's instruction in this letter was probably one of the most important tools a person can ever utilize if they desire to have mental and emotional wellness. No prison, mentally, emotionally, or physically, can dictate your thinking. No situation, thing, or person that you are hanging your hope on will make you satisfied. You alone decide what to think about. Happiness, friends, is an inside job, not an outside situation.

As we near the end of our thirty-one days, mark Paul's timeless advice. Learn what to think. Steer your thoughts. Redirect them a million times if you have to. This is the secret to surviving anything and having contentment in everything.

"After they were severely beaten, they were thrown into prison and the jailer was commanded to guard them securely. So the jailer placed them in the innermost cell of the prison and had their feet bound and chained. Paul and Silas, undaunted, prayed in the middle of the night and sang songs of praise to God, while all the other prisoners listened to their worship." (Acts 16:23–25 TPT)

FURTHER THOUGHTS

- Do your outside circumstances drive your happiness? Why or why not?
- What thoughts can you utilize to interject in your hardest situations right now?

IF AT FIRST YOU DON'T SUCCEED . . .

YOU'VE MADE IT . . . UNTIL the last day anyways. For some of us, committing to thirty-one days of anything is huge. For that, I celebrate you.

I hope that you walk away with some knowledge and understanding to equip you. And while completing the last thirty-one days isn't small by any means, I want to encourage you with this: keep going.

My life has been a process. I'm still learning and applying the same core ideas I've shared with you. Tomorrow isn't day thirty-two for me, but day one yet again.

Keep building on what you've started. Keep kicking down the lies and nurturing the truth of Scripture. Keep praying. Keep fighting. If you do, the unfathomable things that seemed impossible to overcome will finally fall like the Goliath they seem to be.

Here are some verses to encourage your endurance. Please know that I'm rooting for you!

"Patient endurance is what you need now, so that you will

continue to do God's will. Then you will receive all that he has promised." (Hebrews 10:36 NLT)

"As for the rest of you, dear brothers and sisters, never get tired of doing good." (2 Thessalonians 3:13 NLT)

"Let this hope burst forth within you, releasing a continual joy. Don't give up in a time of trouble, but commune with God at all times." (Romans 12:12 TPT)

"If your faith remains strong, even while surrounded by life's difficulties, you will continue to experience the untold blessings of God! True happiness comes as you pass the test with faith, and receive the victorious crown of life promised to every lover of God!" (James 1:12 TPT)

FURTHER THOUGHTS

- How are you in a better place at the end of this devotional than you were at the beginning?
- What are the most important themes from the past month that you will continue to build on as you go from here?
- I'd love to have some feedback. Email me your biggest takeaways from this devo. You can also email some suggestions to help improve this study for the future.

IF YOU'RE A FAN OF THIS BOOK, WILL YOU HELP ME SPREAD THE WORD?

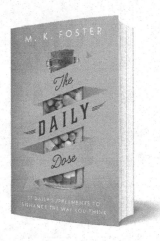

There are several ways you can help me get the word out about the message of this book...

- Post a 5-Star review on Amazon.
- Write about the book on your Facebook, Twitter, Instagram, LinkedIn — any social media you regularly use!
- If you blog, consider referencing the book, or publishing an excerpt from the book with a link back to my website. You have my permission to do this as long as you provide proper credit and backlinks.
- Recommend the book to friends — word-of-mouth is still the most effective form of advertising.
- Purchase additional copies to give away as gifts.

The best way to connect with me is by email:
buildingyourmomentum365@gmail.com

Visit my blog: www.buildingyourmomentum.com